APPLE CIDER VINEGAR

MIGHTY BOOSTER FOR YOUR BEAUTY, HEALTH, AND REJUVENATION

SIMPLE & SMART ACV RECIPES
FOR YOUR SKIN, HAIR & NAILS

Irina K.

CONTENTS

ISBN 978-1-9806-3022-7

DISCLAIMER

PLEASE NOTE THAT ANY TIPS IN THIS BOOK ARE NOT AND SHOULD NOT BE USED TO REPLACE MEDICAL ADVICE FROM A LICENSED PROFESSIONAL. NEITHER THIS BOOK NOR ANY OF THE RECIPES CONTAINED IN THIS BOOK (THE "CONTENT") ARE A SUBSTITUTE FOR MEDICAL ADVICE FROM YOUR PHYSICIAN OR HEALTH ADVICE FROM ANY QUALIFIED HEALTH PROFESSIONAL. YOU SHOULD DISCUSS YOUR PARTICULAR ISSUE(S) OR ANY CONCERNS WITH YOUR OWN PHYSICIAN OR OTHER LICENSED PROFESSIONAL. THE INFORMATION CONTAINED IN THIS BOOK AND/OR OTHERWISE RECEIVED FROM US IS NOT INTENDED TO DIAGNOSE, TREAT, CURE, OR PREVENT ANY DISEASE.

NEITHER THE AUTHOR NOR THE CONTENT PROVIDERS SHALL BE HELD LIABLE OR RESPONSIBLE FOR ANY LOSS, DAMAGE, INJURY, OR ILLNESS SUFFERED BY YOU AND/OR CAUSED OR ALLEGEDLY CAUSED DIRECTLY OR INDIRECTLY BY ANY TREATMENT, ACTION, OR USE OF ANY OF THE CONTENT OR FOR ANY MISUNDERSTANDING OR MISUSE OF THE INFORMATION CONTAINED IN THIS BOOK.

INTRODUCTION

Thank you for purchasing the updated version of my book. For the last two years I enriched my experience of using apple cider vinegar (ACV) for health and beauty and decided to share with you some more tips and recipes.

This book contains the best beautifying recipes made with natural ACV for face skin, body skin and shape, hair and nail care. The most of recipes are quite simple to prepare and use, but, nevertheless, very effective, especially when used regularly and in accordance with the given instructions.

We are all creations of our Mother Nature. Nature has provided us with everything needed to keep up with our health and beauty. There are so many wonderful and simple recipes that use a variety of natural resources. So why use artificially created means, which contain a tremendous number of chemical components that affect us and nature in a negative way? Yes, maybe the natural remedies could require more time for their preparation and use in comparison with the ready-made synthetic products. However, the long-lasting result of their use is also much better, without side-effects, if applied properly. Also, natural remedies are safe for the environment that is a huge advantage. I think that makes it worth to apply some extra effort. The benefits will pay it off with interest!

Natural ACV is a truly unique product, known since ancient times and being one of the most popular folk remedies used around the world today for the treatment and prevention of various diseases and ailments. Its effectiveness is confirmed by its use over centuries in various countries – a time-tested remedy.

Natural ACV is vinegar made by fermentation of apple juice, without chemical additives. Such vinegar contains more than 60 organic compounds, 16 amino acids, vitamins (A, B1, B2, B3, B5, B6, B7, C, E), acids (acetic, malic, citric, lactic, oxalic), micro- and macro elements (potassium, copper, silicon, magnesium, calcium, iron, sodium, phosphorus, sulfur), and enzymes. It has so many benefits for our bodies both inside and out. Natural ACV has pronounced healing, regenerating, soothing, cleansing, anti-bacterial, and anti-microbial effects. ACV has a whole arsenal of useful properties for the skin; it acts as a soft peel, helps to remove dead skin cells, evens out skin tone, and helps to get rid of age spots and acne scars. Due to pronounced antiseptic effect, ACV relieves inflammation, accelerates the disappearance of bruises and pimples, heals minor damages like scratches, insect bites, etc. ACV is also a great aftershave and post-epilation/depilation cure that eliminates ingrown hair, razor rash, itchiness, red bumps, pimples, and spots. It also smooths fine lines and wrinkles, improves skin elasticity, restores the natural acidic environment on the skin surface, reduces stretch marks. ACV is also effective against cellulite, especially when combined with physical activity and a healthy diet. Through active fruit acids, apple cider vinegar speeds up the metabolism in problem areas, destroying cellulite deposits, splitting fats, and helping to remove them from the body.

This amazing natural remedy has been successfully used for the recovery and preservation of youth and beauty, as well as in cooking and as an ecological means to keep your home clean. In other words, natural ACV is a real treasure trove of useful ingredients for the human body and home, a fact that explains its growing popularity worldwide.

It is possible to write whole volumes about ACV; its history, how to obtain and use it in treatment, cosmetology, cooking, cleaning, and everyday life, because this topic is so extensive and interesting. The purpose of this book is to describe specific and effective recipes using ACV as a home cosmetic product for skin, hair, and nail care. All the recipes in this book have been tested by me personally, as well as by many of my relatives and friends, with stable and positive results. A noticeable positive effect can occur within a week or two after regular use of ACV according to recipes below. The most natural means work effectively with long and regular use with respect to the guidelines given. The longer and more regularly you use ACV in the right dosage, the greater the benefits.

The sharp smell of ACV quickly disappears within a few minutes after use, so you need not worry that your house or your body will exude the smell of vinegar.

I personally discovered ACV more than eight years ago and since then I have been using it; at least one liter of this wonderful substance is always in my house. How did I start to use ACV? It began when I was faced with a very unpleasant problem – dandruff. I always trusted nature and preferred natural beautifying and wellness means, so I started to search for the solution among folk remedies. During my search, I came across descriptions of some dandruff treatments that use natural apple cider vinegar. I decided to try these remedies and did not regret it; the dandruff quickly disappeared after 5 or 6 applications of ACV, and the general condition of my hair improved: it became softer, easy to comb and got more shine. I was more than satisfied. After that I started learning more about ACV and various recipes and remedies based on it for maintenance and improvement of health, youth, and beauty.

Natural ACV also has powerful anti-aging properties, which were known as far back as ancient times.

PLEASE READ THE **'IMPORTANT INFORMATION'** SECTION BEFORE YOU START TO USE THE ACV RECIPES. IT IS VERY IMPORTANT!

I hope you will love my recipes and find them useful. I wish natural ACV will become your loyal companion and that your life will be full of health, harmony, and beauty!

I would be happy to receive your feedback and know what you liked most in this book. Enjoy the reading!

IMPORTANT INFORMATION

The internal application of ACV is useful only in case of absence of contraindications to this product. If you have any serious diseases or doubts concerning the consequences of ACV use, consult your doctor before starting to use it.

Be aware that the acidity of the store-bought ACV (4-6%) is usually higher than the acidity of the homemade version (3%). When you use the store-bought ACV, remember that it should be diluted with water in a bit larger proportions than indicated in the recipes for homemade vinegar. This book contains the proportions for using the store-bought ACV.

Natural ACV is suitable for any skin type, but it should be applied with caution if you have very sensitive skin, as it can cause some irritation.

I advise you to use a drinking straw while consuming diluted ACV to protect your tooth enamel against the vinegar's acids. If used frequently, apple cider vinegar, like any other acid, may adversely affect the condition of your tooth enamel. If you don't have a drinking straw on hand, then simply rinse your mouth with fresh water right after finishing your drink.

It is better to store ACV in a tinted glass bottle. Glass is an ideal material for product storage, especially for acids. The tinted glass protects products against sunlight that can degrade the product's quality.

The vinegar should be stored in a dark place at room temperature. No need to keep it in the fridge. The best place is a grocery cupboard located away from any heat sources. It is very important to store ACV in a tightly closed bottle so it does not evaporate. Plastic and metallic containers are not suitable for vinegar storage. The plastic ones could start to corrode and to secrete harmful substances and the metallic ones could start to oxidize because of the vinegar's influence, thereby worsening the vinegar's quality.

HOW TO DISTINGUISH NATURAL APPLE CIDER VINEGAR

Ideally, it is better to use homemade ACV. Today we can find a lot of free information about how to make ACV by ourselves. If you do not have the time or desire to prepare homemade apple cider vinegar, you can always use a purchased version instead. The best choice would be organic ACV made from organically grown apples that contain absolutely no additives.

How to distinguish natural ACV from synthetic ones? There are several characteristics allowing you to distinguish natural ACV from synthetic kinds:

1. The label of natural ACV should indicate: *"Apple cider vinegar"* or *"Pure apple cider vinegar"*. If the vinegar contains: *"Acetic acid 9%, flavor, color ... etc."* – it is not a natural product, but a synthetic one, and it does not possess the useful properties that natural apple cider vinegar does.
2. The acidity of natural ACV is 3-6%. The acidity of synthetic vinegar is 9%.
3. Natural ACV may contain minor sediments of natural origin; this is a normal occurrence.
4. The price of natural ACV is usually higher than the price of synthetic ACV.

A LITTLE BIT OF HISTORY

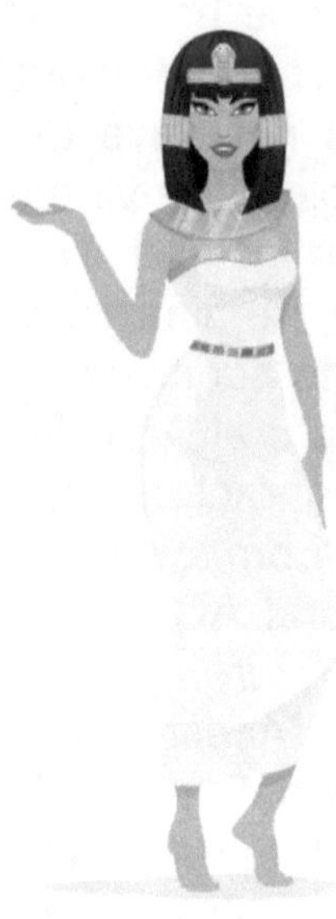

People knew how to make ACV even thousands of years ago; various documents from different ages and countries confirm this. In ancient Babylon, Egypt, and Assyria ACV was used for the treatment of many diseases. During military campaigns, Roman legionaries took with them diluted apple cider vinegar, since it perfectly quenched their thirst and also served as a disinfectant for wounds and infections. In Chinese medicine, ACV has also held a place of honor; Chinese Aesculapius used it in acupuncture treatments. In the Old Testament, apple cider vinegar is referred to as an indispensable product, which was used as a spice and remedy in almost every home. Also, ACV served as an effective anti-fungal and anti-inflammatory agent which helped to get rid of lice. In ancient Egypt, ACV was used by women as a major beauty product for hair, face, body, and skin care. It is known that the legendary

Egyptian queen Cleopatra used vinegar to preserve her health and beauty. Cleopatra took baths with rose oil, after which servants rubbed a mixture of olive oil and apple cider vinegar, in equal proportions, into the Queen's skin, so Cleopatra's beautiful skin could retain its elasticity and suppleness. There is also a legend connecting apple cider vinegar with the name of the great queen. It says that once, during dinner, Cleopatra bet with her beloved Mark Antony claiming that she could eat dishes for ten million sesterces. Grandees surrounding the Queen were stunned about such a claim, since even they, who got used to throwing their money around, couldn't imagine that it would be possible to eat dishes totaling such a huge sum during one dinner; actually, it was the sum the ordinary Egyptian merchant earned in 5-6 years. Within view of all guests, Cleopatra threw several pearls estimated at ten million sesterces in a cup filled with vinegar and began to indulge in serene fun. While the feast was occurring, the pearls completely dissolved in the vinegar. Cleopatra diluted the vinegar-pearl solvent with clear water and drank the precious drink worth ten million sesterces, having proved once again her finesse and originality.

In the 13th century, Western Europe had already known the industrial production of vinegar, but for a long-time people did not understand the whole process of turning wine into vinegar. In the 19th century, English poet D. Byron used a so-called "peasant diet" for weight loss. He drank apple cider vinegar, diluting it with water, and ate black crackers. Extant data reported that, as a result of this diet, the lord grew considerably thin and, according to his personal statement, began to feel much better.

The American doctor of medicine and naturopath, D.S. Jarvis, considered apple cider vinegar to be one of the most useful products in the world and recommended to accept it for treatment of various diseases, including chronic ones. Dr. Jarvis also recommended drinking diluted ACV for weight loss. The Academician Boris Bolotov, who is often called the Ukrainian magician and who discovered a way that made it possible for anyone to live for up to 150 years old, also considered apple cider vinegar as one of the most important natural means of maintaining health, youth, and beauty. Boris Bolotov described his own method of ACV preparation, as well as many recipes for its use for healing and regeneration.

FACE & BODY MASSAGE LINES

When you apply a mask or tonic on your face, or use a face or body scrub, or do some sort of massaging, it is better that your hand movements follow massage lines on your face and body. This will highly improve the therapeutic and beautifying effect of your procedures.

Massage lines are the lines of the least skin stretching. Following these lines during the facial treatments helps to improve the facial oval, makes facial features more expressive and beautiful, improves the skin color and texture, and helps to get rid of wrinkles and pimples. On the contrary, not following the facial massage lines can make it all worse. Edemas could appear on the face, the skin could become loose and covered with wrinkles. Following the massage lines during the body treatment is also important. It improves lymph flow and skin elasticity. Therefore, remember that following the massage lines is very important and highly beneficial. What are these lines? Please look at the pictures below:

FACIAL MASSAGE LINES

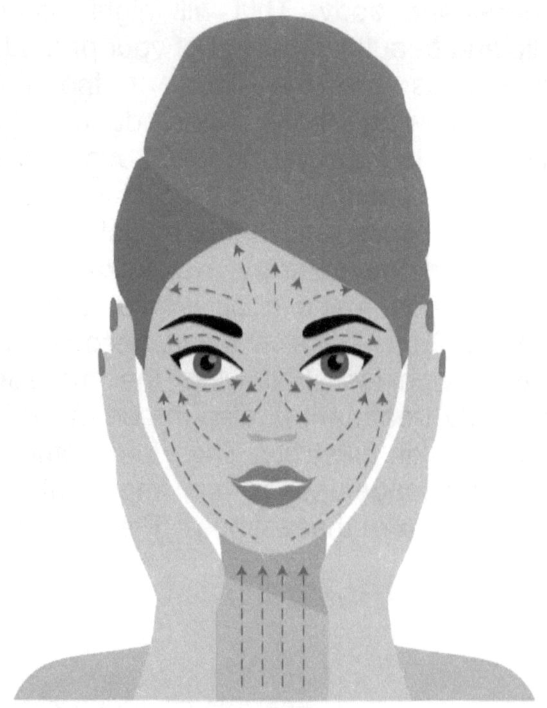

BODY MASSAGE LINES

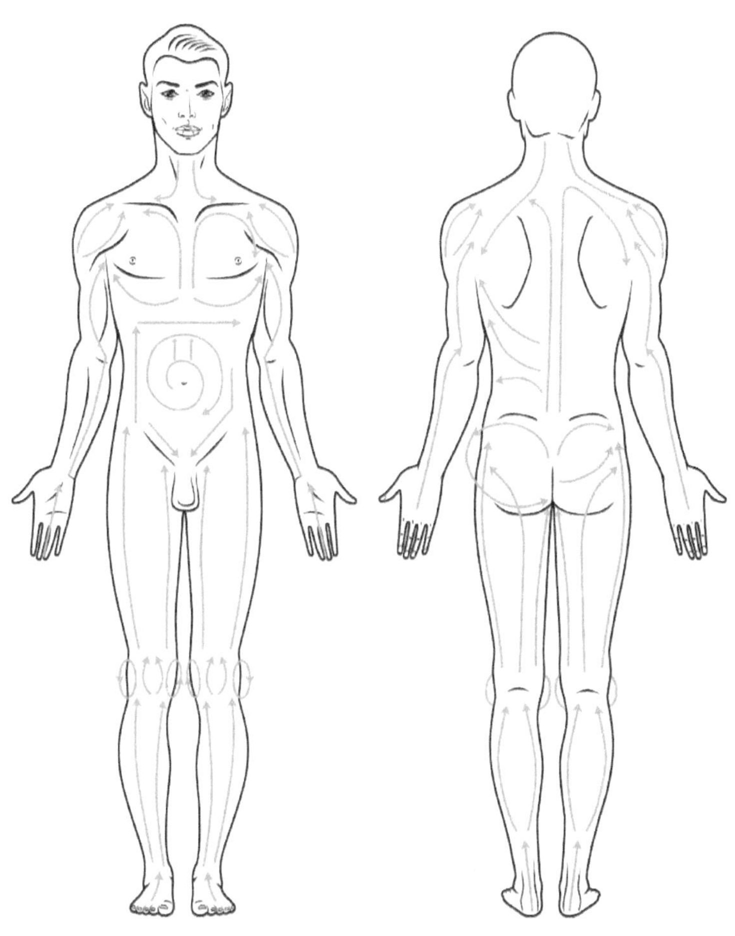

FACIAL CARE RECIPES

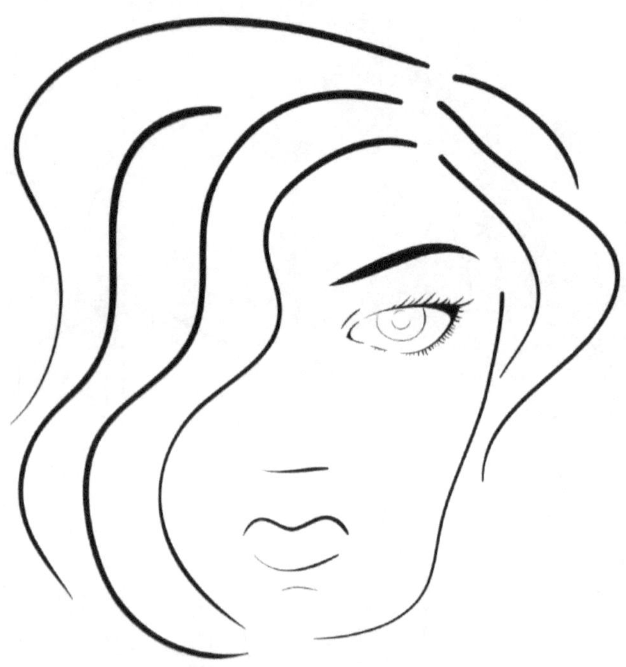

ACV PEEL FOR CLEAN, EVEN AND VELVETY SKIN – THE OVERVIEW

Peel with ACV is an effective way to improve the condition and appearance of your face skin. Face peel is considered one of the important steps in skin care routine. Dead skin particles and clogged pores prevents the skin from fully absorb all of the available nutrients containing in masks and creams. In addition, the skin can not "breath" normally that causes its unusual grayness and flabbiness. Natural apple cider vinegar will help to fix this. Peels with ACV are especially useful for problem and oily skin. They gently cleanse the skin, heal acne, and sooth the foci of inflammatory lesions of the face.

Peel with ACV provides plenty of benefits for your face skin:

- ACV kills harmful bacteria and fights acne.
- ACV contains polyphenols, enzymes, and minerals that participate in skin rejuvenation and transformation. ACV peel makes the face look fresh and bright, evens the skin tone, eliminates small wrinkles slowing down the appearance of the new ones.
- Beta-carotene contained in ACV – is a strong antioxidant neutralizing free radicals. ACV antioxidant properties help to prevent early withering of the skin.
- ACV peel gently cleanses the skin, cures acne, and soothes skin inflammation and irritation.
- ACV lightens and reduces pigment spots, improves skin elasticity. Skin becomes perfectly smooth and velvety. ACV contains acetic acid that eliminates black dots and sebaceous filaments.

NOTES:

- Frequency of use: For normal and dry skin it is enough to use ACV peel once per week; for oily skin it is ok to use it twice per week.
- Peel with ACV can cause short-term redness of the skin. It is a normal reaction, but, it is better to wait a couple of hours before going outside, especially during the hot summer or cold winter time. To protect your skin after peel, use a suitable sunscreen during summer and nourishing cream during winter.
- Wait for 3-4 days after peeling before using face scrubs – let your skin to recover.

ACV peel is a way to an ideal and velvety skin. After a few procedures you will notice a rejuvenating effect, more clean pores, and more fresh face tone. Dedicate 10 to 15 minutes a week for ACV peel and you will not regret it!

PEEL # 1: "FRUIT ALLSORTS"
(FOR OILY & PROBLEM SKIN)

This peel with fruit juices greatly improves the condition of the problem and oily skin, helps to get rid of acne, and remove shine & oily glare from face.

Ingredients:
o   *1 tsp. of ACV;*
o   *1 tsp. of fresh orange juice;*
o   *1 tsp. of blackcurrant juice without additives;*
o   *1 tsp. of corn oil.*

How to proceed:

- Mix all the ingredients together.

- Apply evenly on your clean face with a cotton pad or a soft facial sponge.

- Wait for five minutes. *In case of unpleasant burning feeling, rinse the mixture off with clean warm water and in the future always dilute it with water in a proportion optimal for you.*

- To accelerate the exfoliation of the stratum corneum, do a small massage with a soft face sponge. Moisten the sponge in a mixture and gently rub your skin along the massage lines as shown in the picture in the section FACE & BODY MASSAGE LINES.

- Rinse your face with warm water.

- Apply a moisturizing face cream.

NOTE: Peel with ACV and fruit acids can cause unnatural redness of the skin due to the active effect of acetic and ascorbic acids. You should not worry about this, the redness will disappear within a couple of hours.

PEEL # 2: MILK & FRUIT & ACV
(FOR ALL SKIN TYPES)

This recipe is suitable for all skin types. Helps to fight acne, sebaceous filaments, comedones, and inflammatory processes. Milk & fruit peel with ACV is a precious find for your face.

Ingredients:
- *1 tsp. of ACV;*
- *1 tbsp. of fresh orange juice;*
- *1 tbsp. of chilled whole milk.*

How to proceed:
- Mix milk and orange juice. The milk will have white flakes.
- Add ACV and thoroughly mix.
- Apply evenly on your clean face with a cotton pad or a soft facial sponge.
- Wait for five to seven minutes.
- Rinse your face with room temperature water.
- Apply a moisturizing face cream.

PEEL # 3: WINE & ACV
(FOR ALL SKIN TYPES)

Red wine increases the blood circulation and strengthens the blood vessels increasing their elasticity. This procedure considerably improves the complexion, rejuvenates and smooths the skin. To achieve the desired result after peel, use the natural wine only. If it contains a large number of chemical dyes, it can provoke some irritation or allergic reaction.

Ingredients:
- *1 tsp. of ACV;*
- *3 tsp. of dry red wine.*

How to proceed:
- Mix all the ingredients together.
- Apply evenly on your clean face with a cotton pad or a soft facial sponge.
- Wait for two minutes.
- Apply the mixture on your face the second time (do not rinse off the first layer).
- Wait for two minutes.
- Apply the mixture on your face the third time.
- Wait for three minutes.
- Rinse your face with cool water.
- Apply a moisturizing face cream.

PEEL # 4: "GOMMAGE"
(FOR ALL SKIN TYPES)

The face gommage carefully cleans the skin pores from any kind of contamination. It can be used even for the most delicate, thin, or sensitive skin.

Ingredients:
- *1 tsp. of ACV;*
- *half of an apple;*
- *3 tsp. of natural olive or almond oil.*

How to proceed:
- Mash the apple in a blender or using a grater. You should get a puree consistency.
- Add ACV and oil.
- Thoroughly mix all the ingredients together.
- Apply evenly on your clean face with a cotton pad or a soft facial sponge.
- Wait for five to seven minutes to let it dry.
- Gently massage your skin with fingertips to make the gommage "roll" off the skin.
- Rinse your face with water at a comfortable temperature.
- Apply a moisturizing face cream.

PEEL # 5: FACIAL COMPRESS TO RENEW SKIN, REMOVE KERATINIZED DEAD SKIN CELLS AND PIGMENT SPOTS (FOR ALL SKIN TYPES)

This procedure helps to clean your face, get rid of old skin cells, nourish your skin with useful substances and oxygen. It also helps to get rid of pigmentary and black spots. Your face will become more healthy, fresh, soft, and fine. It is recommended to use this compress once per week.

Ingredients:
- *3 tbsp. of ACV;*
- *half-liter of water.*

How to proceed:
- Clean your face with your favorite cleanser (alcohol-free).

- Soak a small towel in very warm but not hot water, gently wring it out, and put it on your face for a few minutes. It is needed to open skin pores for more active absorption of nutrients contained in ACV.

- Take a small linen cloth or towel, soak it in warm diluted ACV (3 tablespoons of ACV + a half-liter of water), gently wring it out, and put it on your face.

- Get in a comfortable and/or relaxing pose (it is better to lie down) and hold the compress on your face for 5-7 minutes.

- Remove the towel and rinse your face with clean, warm water.

- Wipe your skin with gentle massaging movements, using a wet towel to remove old skin cells. Don't wipe your face with a dry towel because it can injure your skin, which is sensitive after steam.

- Let it dry on its own.
- When the skin is dry, apply a cream suitable for your skin type.

FACIAL SCRUB (FOR ALL SKIN TYPES)

It is recommended to use this scrub once per week. This scrub cleans skin pores, removes old skin cells, disinfects, and improves your skin blood flow. After this procedure, your skin will become more healthy, smooth, fresh, soft, and silky. The natural ACV is also highly effective against pigmentary and black spots. Remember that you shouldn't use scrubs often during the summer time, since they can provoke appearances of age spots. After scrubbing in the summer time, be sure to use sunscreen to protect your skin and to avoid age spots.

Ingredients:
- *1 tbsp. of ACV;*
- *1 tbsp. of honey;*
- *1 tsp. of fine table salt or sea salt (better choice).*

How to proceed:
- Thoroughly mix all the ingredients together.
- Apply evenly the resulting mixture on your face, neck, and decollete.
- <u>Gently</u> massage your skin for 3-5 minutes following the massage lines as shown in the picture in the section FACE & BODY MASSAGE LINES.
- Wash the mixture away with warm water.
- Rinse your face with cool water (to close skin pores).
- Apply a suitable face cream.

MASK FOR OILY, COMBINATION, AND PROBLEM SKIN

This mask regulates the functioning of sebaceous glands, minimizes skin pores, eliminates oily shine, gives skin a perfect matte finish, and helps to eliminate acne and pigmentary spots. It is recommended to use this mask 1-2 times per week.

Ingredients:
- *4 tbsp. of ACV;*
- *2 tsp. of warm honey;*
- *2 tbsp. of oatmeal (ground into fine oat flour).*

How to proceed:
- Thoroughly mix all the ingredients together.
- Apply evenly the resulting substance to your face, neck, and decollete.
- Wait for 20-30 minutes.
- Wash the mixture away with warm water.
- Rinse your face with cool water or a cool decoction of chamomile (to close skin pores).

MASK FOR DRY AND NORMAL SKIN

This mask moisturizes and nourishes the skin. It also helps to get rid of pigmentary and black spots. It is recommended to use this mask 1-2 times per week.

Ingredients:
- *1 tbsp. of ACV;*
- *1 egg yolk;*
- *1 tbsp. of sour cream or Greek yogurt;*
- *1 tbsp. of honey.*

How to proceed:

- Thoroughly mix all the ingredients together until obtaining a homogeneous mask.

- Apply evenly the mixture to your clean face, neck, and decollete.

- Wait for 15-20 minutes.

- Wash the mask away with warm water.

- Rinse your skin with cool water (to close skin pores).

REJUVENATION AND WHITENING MASK – FOR EVEN TONE WITHOUT BLACK AND PIGMENT SPOTS (FOR ALL SKIN TYPES)

This mask provides a rejuvenating, bleaching, toning, and smoothing effect for your skin. It also removes pigmentary and black spots.This mask can be used for hands. It is recommended to use this mask 1-2 times per week.

Ingredients:
- *1 tbsp. of ACV;*
- *1 egg yolk;*
- *1 tbsp. of olive oil;*
- *3 tbsp. of peeled grated cucumber.*

How to proceed:
- Mix until obtaining a homogeneous mask.
- Apply evenly the mask onto your clean face, neck, and decollete.
- Wait for 20-30 minutes.
- Wash the substance away with warm water.
- Rinse your skin with cool water or a cool decoction of chamomile (to close skin pores).

MASK FOR ALL SKIN TYPES

This mask moisturizes, nourishes your skin with useful substances, smooths out fine wrinkles, improves skin tone and texture, helps to eliminate pigmentary spots. It is recommended to use this mask 1-2 times per week.

Ingredients:
- *1 tbsp. of ACV;*
- *1 egg yolk;*
- *2 tbsp. of cottage cheese (medium-fat);*
- *1 tbsp. of honey.*

How to proceed:

- Mix until obtaining a homogeneous mask.

- Apply evenly the mask onto your clean face.

- Wait for 15-20 minutes.

- Wash the mask away with warm water.

- Rinse your skin with cool water (to close skin pores).

FACIAL TONER FOR SILKY SKIN WITHOUT BLACK AND PIGMENT SPOTS
(FOR ALL SKIN TYPES)

It is useful to wipe your skin with this toner 1-2 times per day, in the morning and in the evening before going to bed. After treatment, your skin is cleaned, disinfected, and enriched with useful nutrients. Also, the skin becomes more elastic and velvety and develops a healthier color. It also helps to get rid of pigmentary and black spots.

Ingredients <u>for oily, problematic, normal, and combination skin</u>:
- o   *1 tbsp. of ACV;*
- o   *5 tbsp. of water (pre-boiled or filtered).*

Ingredients <u>for dry, sensitive skin</u>:
- o   *1 tbsp. of ACV;*
- o   *10 tbsp. of water (pre-boiled or filtered).*

How to proceed:
- Mix ACV with water.
- Moisten a cotton ball in the resulting solution.
- <u>Gently</u> wipe your face with sliding movements along massage lines as shown in the picture in the section FACE & BODY MASSAGE LINE. Don't pull the skin under the eyes; just slightly moisten your skin.
- Don't wipe it with a towel, let it air dry by itself.
- When the skin becomes dry, apply a cream suitable for your skin type.

Ingredients <u>for inflamed skin</u>:
- o   *1 tbsp. of ACV;*
- o   *5 tbsp. of water (pre-boiled or filtered).*

How to proceed:

- Mix ACV with water.

- Take a cotton ball and soak it in the toner.

- Apply a cotton ball on the inflamed skin and hold for 1-5 minutes.

- Don't wipe it with a towel, let it air dry by itself.

<u>NOTE</u>: It is better to do this in the evening before going to bed. This procedure will disinfect and heal the skin accelerating its recovery. Be careful and watch for your skin reaction. In case of allergic reaction (extreme redness, itching), rinse your skin with a large amount of warm water and then use moisturizing or baby cream.

COSMETIC ICE WITH ACV FOR FRESH AND BRIGHT FACE WITHOUT SPOTS AND DOTS (FOR ALL SKIN TYPES)

Cosmetic ice with natural ACV works wonders on skin! It tones up the skin and mobilizes its protective properties, strengthens the blood vessels and narrows pores, removes pigmentary and black spots. Also it helps to keep the skin looking young and improves its elasticity, removes small wrinkles and reduces the appearance of deep wrinkles. Dark circles and swellings under the eyes disappear. Use 1-2 cubes daily for your morning and evening beauty ritual. It is a great way to cheer up in the morning.

WARNING: Do not use the cosmetic ice if you have couperose (vascular sprouts), skin inflammation or eczema. Use with caution if you have acne. Wait for 3-4 days after peel before using the cosmetic ice – let your skin to recover.

Ingredients:
- *1 tbsp. of ACV;*
- *200 ml of fresh clean water.*

How to proceed:
- Brew 200 ml of fresh clean water and cool it down.
- Add 1 tbsp. of ACV and mix it.
- Freeze the diluted ACV in the ice cube tray.
- Take 1-2 ice cubes and gently wipe your face skin along the massage lines as shown in the picture in the section FACE & BODY MASSAGE LINES during 1-2 minutes.
- Do not wipe with a towel, let it dry itself.

- Apply your favourite cream.

To make it even more beneficial, you can use a herbal decoction instead of just water. Ice with camomile and calendula is good for all skin types and provides an antiseptic effect. Ice with bidens removes redness, itching, rashes and peeling, normalizes sebum secretions.

Ingredients:
- *1 tbsp. of ACV;*
- *200 ml of fresh clean water;*
- *3 tbsp. of dry camomile or bidens (black jack) or calendula flowers (or their mixture).*

How to proceed:

- Brew 200 ml of fresh clean water and add it to the dry flowers.

- Cool the decoction down.

- Filter the decoction in a kitchen sieve or through gauze.

- Add 1 tbsp. of ACV and mix it.

- Freeze the solution in the ice cube tray.

- Take 1-2 ice cubes and <u>gently</u> wipe your face skin along the massage lines as shown in the picture in the section FACE & BODY MASSAGE LINES during 1-2 minutes.

- Do not wipe with a towel, let it dry itself.

- Apply your favourite cream.

BODY CARE RECIPES

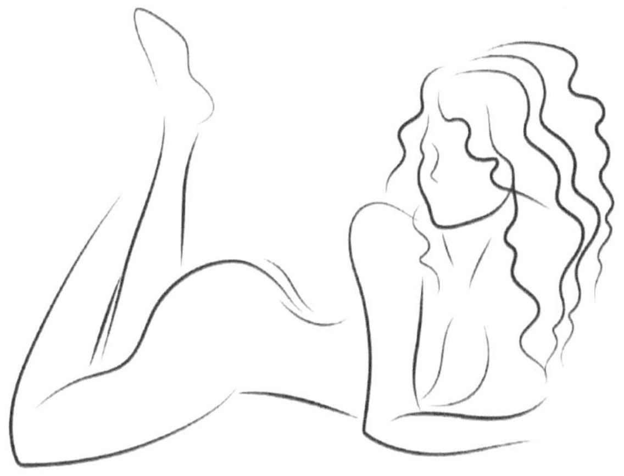

BODY SCRUBS

These scrubs are perfect for cleaning and smoothing the skin, healing micro damaged skin and improving blood circulation. Also, it helps to get rid of ingrown hair and shaving rash. If you use these scrubs regularly, your skin will become smoother, more elastic, and its color and general condition will improve. It is recommended to use these scrubs 1-2 times per week.

Advice: during the massage, it is better to follow the body massage lines as shown in the picture in the section FACE & BODY MASSAGE LINES. This will improve the therapeutic effect of your massage.

Recipe # 1:

Ingredients:
- *3 tbsp. of ACV;*
- *3 tbsp of honey;*
- *3 tsp. of fine or coarse table salt (the salt crystals should not be too big) or sea salt (better choice).*

How to proceed:

- Thoroughly mix all the ingredients together until obtaining a homogeneous mass.

- Apply evenly the mixture onto your body skin, <u>gently</u> massaging it in a circular motion.

- Wash the scrub away with warm water.

- Rinse your skin with cool water (to close skin pores).

- Apply your favourite doby cream/lotion/milk.

<u>Recipe # 2:</u>

Ingredients:
- *3 tbsp. of ACV;*
- *3 tbsp of sour cream or Greek yogurt;*
- *3 tsp. of fine or coarse table salt (the salt crystals should not be too big) or sea salt (better choice).*

How to proceed:
- Thoroughly mix all the ingredients together until obtaining a homogeneous mass.
- Apply evenly the mixture onto your body skin, <u>gently</u> massaging it in a circular motion.
- Wash the scrub away with warm water.
- Rinse your skin with cool water (to close skin pores).
- Apply your favourite doby cream/lotion/milk.

DAILY AFTER SHOWER MASSAGE

This procedure cleans the skin, restores its acidity, disinfects it by removing harmful skin micro-organisms, improves blood circulation, skin tone and texture. Also, it is an efficient remedy against ingrown hair and shaving rash.

It is better to use a sponge made from natural materials, such as luffa or rami. Tourkish kese glove would be another great choice for this procedure. It is 100% natural bath glove that effectively removes dead skin cells from the body, gently cleanses the skin, opens the pores and improves blood circulation.

Ingredients:
- o   *1 tbsp. of ACV;*
- o   *1 cup of warm water.*

How to proceed:
- Take a shower.
- Mix ACV and water.
- Soak a soft sponge or towel in a solution of ACV.
- <u>Gently</u> massage your body following the body massage lines as shown in the picture in the section FACE & BODY MASSAGE LINES. (This will improve the therapeutic effect of your massage).
- Rinse your skin with water at a comfortable temperature.

TONIC MASSAGING

Such massaging disinfects the skin, stimulates blood circulation, restores the natural skin acidity, provides a powerful anti-aging effect, heals after shaving rash and reduces ingrown hairs. It is suggested to massage daily, especially in the morning, as it will energize you for the whole day.

The optimum time for massaging is five to seven minutes. It is not necessary to rinse your body after this or to wipe it with a towel. It is better to let your body air dry at room temperature – to extend the beneficial impact of ACV on your skin.

It is better to use a sponge made from natural materials, such as luffa or rami. Tourkish kese glove would be another great choice for this procedure.

Ingredients:
- *2 tbsp. of ACV;*
- *2 tbsp. of salt (better to use sea salt);*
- *1 liter of water at a room temperature.*

How to proceed:
- Take a shower.
- Mix ACV, salt, and water.
- Moisten a soft sponge or towel in the mixture.
- Rub your body with energetic circular motions in a bottom-up way, starting with legs.

Advice: during the massage, it is better to follow the body massage lines as shown in the picture in the section FACE & BODY MASSAGE LINES. This will improve the therapeutic effect of your massage.

RECIPE FOR CLEANING
AND NOURISHING THE BODY SKIN

This procedure will clean and disinfect your skin, enrich it with nutrients and leave it delicate, fresh, elastic and fragrant (if you use an essential oil). It also helps to get rid of ingrown hair and shaving rash.

Ingredients:
- *2 tsp. of ACV;*
- *½ cup of millet and oat flakes;*
- *2-3 tbsp. of sea salt or rock-salt;*
- *1 tbsp. of sour cream or Greek yogurt;*
- *3-4 tbsp. of oil (pure olive oil is the best choice);*
- *1 egg yolk;*
- *1 tbsp. of honey;*
- *several drops of sage, propolis or peppermint tincture or your favourite essential oil.*

How to proceed:
- Grind salt, millet and oat flakes in a coffee grinder or a suitable blender.

- Add the other ingredients and thoroughly mix it all together.

- Take a shower or bath.

- Apply the mixture onto your wet body, including the face and the neck.

- <u>Gently</u> massage your skin in a circular motion for between five to ten minutes.

- Wash off with warm water.

Advice: during the massage, it is better to follow the body massage lines as shown in the picture in the section FACE & BODY MASSAGE LINES. This will improve the therapeutic effect of your massage.

USEFUL BODY IRRIGATIONS WITH ACV, SALT, AND MELTED WATER

Try these very useful skin irrigations with melt-water, ACV and sea salt. Melt-water is structured water, i.e. water with a specific structure, very similar to the liquid in our bodies. Such water provides tones of benefits to our health. Such irrigations are especially useful in the morning: the cool water will energize you, and the ACV and sea salt will disinfect your skin and create a protective barrier on it. This cool solution helps to close the skin pores and positively affects the vessels. Fresh melt water increases the body's resistance to infection, gives a lot of strength, energy, and vitality.

Ingredients:
- *2-3 tbsp. of ACV;*
- *1 tsp. of sea salt;*
- *1 liter of clean water.*

How to proceed:
- Freeze 1 liter of clean water.
- Defrost the ice at a room temperature.
- Add ACV and sea salt in the resulting water.
- Mix all together well.
- Take a shower or bath.
- Apply the resulting solution onto your skin in small portions and massage it all over your body, including the neck and face.

Advice: during the massage, it is better to follow the body massage lines as shown in the picture in the section FACE & BODY MASSAGE LINES. This will improve the therapeutic effect of the procedure.

ACV AGAINST INGROWN HAIR

Natural ACV is a very effective natural remedy against ingrown hair. ACV contains organic acids which soften the upper layer of the epidermis, exfoliate dead cells, disinfect, remove toxins, and increase cellular immunity. If you have a problem of ingrown hair, try this recipe. You can use such wiping for any area of your body: legs, armpits, bikini area – but **be very careful with the bikini area: do not allow ACV to come into contact with mucous membranes**.

This procedure acts like a light peel due to the presence of organic acids helping the ingrown hairs break through the skin. It also cleans and disinfects the skin, removes irritation, heals small wounds reducing the appearance of red spots, bumps, pimples and rash, and eliminates pigmentary spots. You will see a noticeable result in just about a week of a daily application: your skin will become more even, smooth and silky with less of ingrown hairs. The regular use helps to get rid of ingrown hair at all.

This procedure can be done once or twice per day, in the morning and in the evening. To avoid irritation, <u>do not apply this right after your hair removal</u>.

Ingredients:
- *2 parts of ACV (for example 2 tbsp.);*
- *1 part of clean water (for example 1 tbsp.).*

How to proceed:

- Dilute ACV in water in 2:1 proportion.

- Wipe your skin with diluted ACV 15 minutes before taking a shower or bath. For wiping, you can use cotton pads or a soft bath sponge. Do not rub your skin, just wipe it with enough pressure and be sure that the whole area with ingrown hair is moistened with ACV.

NOTE: Right after use you can feel a light burning sensation that is ok, but if the feeling is highly uncomfortable, wash out the ACV with clean water immediately and use ACV with more water in the future.

If you have thick hair and your skin is not sensitive, you can try to use undiluted ACV, but be careful, especially with the bikini area.

NATURAL DEODORANT

After taking a shower or a bath, wipe dry armpits and lubricate them with undiluted ACV. Thanks to its anti-bacterial effect, ACV kills bacteria causing the unpleasant smell of sweat. If possible, repeat this procedure several times a day. The sharp smell of ACV disappears quickly, so don't worry that you will smell as ACV.

TREATMENT FOR ROUGH SKIN ON FEET

Even after only three such baths with a small-time interval, the skin on your feet will become noticeably softer and your nails will acquire a healthier color and shine. This procedure softens the cuticle and facilitates its removal. Also, ACV is highly effective against toenail fungus, reduces sweating and deodorizes your feet.

It is recommended to use this bath solutions one or two times per week.

Ingredients:
- *1 cup of ACV (200 ml);*
- *1-2 liters of warm water.*

How to proceed:

- Pour 1-2 liters of warm water into a suitable container.

- Add ACV and mix well.

- Immerse your feet into this solution.

- Wait for approximately 15 minutes.

- Do not rinse, dry with a towel.

- Lubricate the skin with moisturizing cream (in summer) or nourishing cream (in winter).

BATH TO MAKE YOUR FEET SKIN GENTLE AND SOFT

This bath helps to soften the calluses and the rough skin (corns) on the feet quickly and effectively. You can do this procedure every day. Very soon the skin of your feet will become like a baby's skin – smooth and velvety. Also, it softens the cuticle and facilitates its removal. The toenails will also gain a healthier color and shine. The result could be even better than after visiting a salon! Moreover, the natural ACV reduces sweating and deodorizes your feet. It is better to take such baths in the evening before going to bed.

Ingredients:
o   *1 cup of ACV (200 ml);*
o   *2 liters of warm water;*
o   *2 tbsp. of salt (sea salt is a better choice).*

How to proceed:

- Pour 2 liters of warm (not hot!) water into a vessel.

- Add ACV and salt and mix well.

- Dip your feet into the resulting solution.

- Wait for approximately 10-15 minutes.

- Rub the coarsened skin with a pumice.

- Rinse with water at a comfortable temperature.

- Wipe dry with a towel.

- Grease with a nourishing cream.

- Put on cotton socks to enhance the effect.

BATH WITH ACV

After this your skin will become smooth, soft and velvety. It is recommended to take such bath one or two times per week.

Ingredients:
- *2-3 cups of ACV (400-600 ml);*
- *bath of warm water.*

How to proceed:
- Fill your bath tub with water at a comfortable temperature.
- Add ACV and mix well.
- Use this bath solution for between 15 and 30 minutes.
- You can dip your head in the water – it will positively affect both the skin on your head and your hair.
- There's no need to rinse your skin and hair.
- Wipe dry with a towel.
- <u>Optional</u>: apply your favourite body cream.

MASSAGE AGAINST STRETCH MARKS, SPIDER VEINS AND CELLULITE

This massage will help you to fight stretch marks, spider veins and cellulite. It is also a good remedy against ingrown hair and shaving rash.

Ingredients:
- *1 part of ACV (for example ½ cup);*
- *1 part of clean water (for example ½ cup).*

How to proceed:
- Mix ACV and water.

- Take a hard sponge and moisten it in the mixture (1:1 proportion). Tourkish kese would be a good choice for this procedure.

- Massage gently for between 10 and 15 minutes.

- Rinse your skin with water at a comfortable temperature.

- Dry with a towel.

- <u>Optional</u>: apply your favourite body cream.

<u>Advices</u>:
- During the massage, it is better to follow the body massage lines as shown in the picture in the section FACE & BODY MASSAGE LINES. This will improve the therapeutic effect of your massage.
- Whilst doing the massage, plug the drain hole to avoid draining away the ACV solution. Immerse your feet into this mixture during the procedure and they will gain many benefits: the feet skin will become softer and the toenails will gain a healthier color and shine.

- If you have sensitive skin, massage in this way once a week.
- For normal skin it is good to carry out this procedure every day. You can even try to do this twice a day – in the morning and in the evening.
- The frequency of this procedure depends on your skin type and on your willingness. Watch the reaction of your skin, it will help to determine the ideal frequency of the massage.

ANTI-CELLULITE MASSAGE

This procedure effectively fights cellulite, nourishes the skin and improves its tone and elasticity.

Ingredients:
o   *3 parts of ACV (for example 1.5 cups);*
o   *1 part of olive oil or any massage oil (for example ½ cup);*
o   *optional: several drops of citrus essence oil (orange, grape, lemon).*

How to proceed:

- Thoroughly mix ACV and oil.

- Apply this mixture onto your problem areas.

- <u>Vigorously</u> massage with a hard sponge for between 5 to 15 minutes. Tourkish kese would be a good choice for this procedure. Massage your body with <u>energetic circular motions</u>.

- Rinse your skin with water at a comfortable temperature.

- Dry with a towel.

- <u>Optional</u>: apply your favourite body cream.

<u>Advices</u>:
- During the massage, it is better to follow the body massage lines as shown in the picture in the section FACE & BODY MASSAGE LINES. This will improve the therapeutic effect of your massage.
- <u>To gain a quick and noticeable effect</u> it is recommended to make at least 10 daily massages. It is better to do this massage twice a day: in the morning and in the evening.

-   <u>On a regular basis</u> it is better to carry out this massage every other day, once or twice a day.
-   After this anti-cellulite massage, it is useful to take an anti-cellulite bath with ACV (see the recipe below).

51

ANTI-CELLULITE "HONEY+ACV" COCKTAIL

Ingredients:
- *2 tbsp. of ACV;*
- *2 tbsp. of natural honey;*
- *1-2 tbsp. of warm water.*

How to proceed:

- Thoroughly mix ACV, honey, and water.

- Apply this mixture onto your problem areas.

- <u>Vigorously</u> massage your body for between 5 and 10 minutes with your hands or a hard sponge or towel. Tourkish kese would be another good choice for this procedure.

- <u>To enhance the result</u>, after your massage you can wrap your body with plastic food wrap and put on warm clothes or lie under a blanket for 30 minutes. During this waiting time is it useful to drink a warm green tea or an herbal decoction (linden, rosehip, etc.), it helps to enhance the detoxification process.

- Wash off with warm water.

- Finally, rinse your body with cool water (to calm down your skin after the massage).

- Dry with a towel.

- <u>Optional</u>: Apply your favorite moisturizing or anti-cellulite cream.

<u>Advice</u>: During the massage, it is better to follow the body massage lines as shown in the picture in the section FACE & BODY MASSAGE LINES. This will improve the therapeutic effect of your massage.

ANTI-CELLULITE BATH WITH ACV

This bath helps to fight cellulite and stimulates the removal of toxins. One course – 10 baths every other day. Then take a one-week break.

Ingredients:
- *½ liter of ACV;*
- *½ kilo of sea salt;*
- *bath of warm water (about 37-38 degrees by Celsius).*

How to proceed:
- Fill your bath tub with water. It should not be hot or cold, but comfortable for you.
- Add ACV and sea salt into the bath and mix well.
- Use this bath solution for between 15 and 30 minutes.
- **It is also useful to add five to ten drops of any citrus essential oil (orange, grapefruit, lemon, lime, bergamot)** as it helps to regulate the fat metabolism in the body and stimulates the removal of toxins. To dilute oil in the bath, pre-mix it with a bit of sea salt – it spreads oil evenly in the water and avoids the appearance of oily circles on the surface.
- Take the bath for between 15 and 25 minutes.
- After taking the bath do not take a shower, rub your body actively with a towel or a hard sponge.
- Put on a warm bath robe.
- Drink a warm green tea or an herbal decoction (linden, rosehip, etc.).
- After 15 minutes, when you cool down and your skin absorbs useful nutrients, rinse your body with

warm water followed with cool water (to close the skin pores).

- Wipe dry with a towel.

- <u>Optional</u>: apply a moisturizing or an anti-cellulite cream on your skin.

ANTI-CELLULITE COMPRESSES

Ingredients:
- *1 cup of ACV;*
- *1 cup of warm water;*
- *2 tbsp. of honey.*

How to proceed:

- Mix well ACV, honey, and water.

- Take a gauze (folded in 3-5 layers) or a thin towel and impregnate it with the solution.

- Wrap the problem areas and cover with plastic food wrap (you should feel comfortable, so don't make it too tight).

- To enhance the result, put on warm trousers or lie under a blanket and wait 1 to 1.5 hours.

- During this waiting time is it useful to drink a warm green tea or an herbal decoction (linden, rosehip, etc.), it helps to enhance the detoxification process.

- Wash your skin with warm water.

- Finally, rinse it with cool or cold water (depends on your experience with pouring cold water) — to close the skin pores and improve blood circulation.

- Optional: apply your favourite cream (anti-cellulite for a better result).

ANTI-CELLULITE DOUGH WITH ACV

Ingredients:
- *1 part of ACV (for example 1 cup);*
- *1 part of honey (for example 1 cup);*
- *flour.*

How to proceed:

- Mix ACV and honey in equal proportions.

- Gradually add a bit of flour (1 cup or more) – you should get a soft and elastic dough.

- Form dough flats, put them on the problem areas and fasten with plastic food wrap.

- To enhance the result, put on warm clothes or lie under a blanket.

- During this waiting time is it useful to drink a warm green tea or an herbal decoction (linden, rosehip, etc.), it helps to enhance the detoxification process.

- Wait for 1.5 to 2 hours.

- Remove the compress and rinse your skin with water at a comfortable temperature.

- Optional: apply a moisturizing or anti-cellulite cream to your skin.

ANTI-CELLULITE WRAPS

Ingredients:
- *1 part of ACV (for example 1 cup);*
- *1 part of warm water (for example 1 cup).*

How to proceed:

- Mix ACV with clean warm water in equal proportions.

- Take a small towel or a sponge, moisten it in the ACV solution and rub your skin firmly on the problem areas.

- Do not dry the skin.

- Wrap your body with plastic food wrap, put on warm clothes or just lie under a warm blanket.

- During this waiting time is it useful to drink a warm green tea or an herbal decoction (linden, rosehip, etc.), it helps to enhance the detoxification process.

- Wait for 1 to 1.5 hours.

- Remove the compress and rinse your skin with water at a comfortable temperature.

- Optional: apply a moisturizing or anti-cellulite cream to your skin.

HAND & NAIL CARE RECIPES

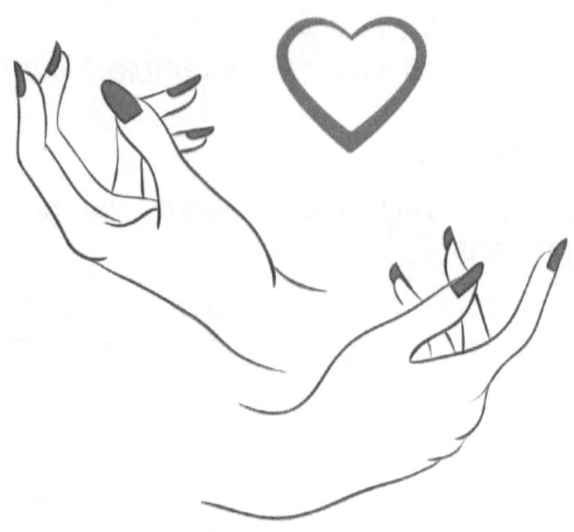

HAND CREAM

It is useful to lubricate the skin on your hands with a cream containing ACV, especially if you have cracked and dry skin. ACV effectively heals it. You can use such cream several times a day. It is especially useful to apply it after dishwashing, cleaning, gardening and washing. With regular use your skin will become smooth, toned, soft and velvety to the touch. Your nails will also gain a healthier color and shine.

Ingredients:
- *1 part of ACV (for example ½ tsp.);*
- *1 part of hand cream (for example ½ tsp.).*

How to proceed:

- Take your regular hand cream and add into it ACV in 1:1 proportion proportions

- Apply the mixture on your hands and nails.

REJUVENATION AND WHITENING MASK
FOR HANDS

This mask provides a rejuvenating, bleaching, toning and smoothing effect for your skin. It is recommended to use this mask one or two times per week.

Ingredients:
- *1 tbsp. of ACV;*
- *1 egg yolk;*
- *1 tsp. of olive oil;*
- *1 tsp. of peeled grated cucumber.*

How to proceed:
- Thoroughly mix all the ingredients until obtaining a homogeneous mass.
- Apply this mixture on your hands.
- Wait for 10 minutes.
- Wash the mask off with warm water.
- Rinse your skin with cool water.

TREATMENT FOR ROUGH SKIN ON HANDS

This treatment makes the skin on your hands noticeably softer. Your nails will acquire a healthier color and shine. It is recommended to use this bath solutions one or two times per week.

Ingredients:
- *½ cup of ACV (100 ml);*
- *1 liter of warm water.*

How to proceed:
- Pour 1 liter of warm water into a suitable container.
- Add ACV to the water.
- Immerse your palms into this solution for between 5 and 15 minutes.
- Do not rinse.
- Dry with a towel.
- Lubricate the skin with moisturizing cream (in summer) or nourishing cream (in winter).

ACV FOR BEAUTIFUL AND HEALTHY NAILS

To keep your nails healthy and beautiful, wipe them periodically with a cotton swab dipped in diluted natural ACV. After doing this your nails will become smoother and will gain a beautiful healthy shine. Also wiping your nails will help to whiten any yellowing and soften cuticles facilitating their removal. This procedure also helps to restore the health and beauty of the nails after being damaged by alkali, for example after washing or dishwashing.

Ingredients:
- *1 part of ACV (for example 1 tsp.);*
- *1 part of hand cream (for example 1 tsp.).*

How to proceed:
- Mix fresh water and ACV in 1:1 proportion.
- Moisten a cotton ball or pad in this solution and wipe your nails.

NAIL-WHITENING BATH WITH ACV

This bath whitens and strengthens your nails and softens the cuticle, facilitating its removal. You can take such bath one or two times a week.

Ingredients:
- *2 tbsp. of ACV;*
- *1 cup of warm water;*
- *5-10 drops of fresh lemon juice.*

How to proceed:

- Mix all the ingredients together.

- Soak your nails in this mixture for 5 to 10 minutes.

- Dry your nails well with a towel or paper napkin.

- Apply nourishing cream with gentle massaging moves.

NAIL-STRENGTHENING BATH WITH ACV

This bath strengthens your nails and softens the cuticle, facilitating its removal. You can take such bath one or two times a week.

Ingredients:
- *2 tbsp. of ACV;*
- *1 cup of warm water;*
- *1 pitch of citric acid OR 1 tsp. of sea salt.*

How to proceed:
- Mix all the ingredients together.
- Soak your nails in this mixture for 5 to 10 minutes.
- Dry your nails well with a towel or paper napkin.
- Apply nourishing cream with gentle massaging moves.

BATH WITH ACV FOR FRAGILE NAILS

This bath helps to strengthen fragile nails and fights against splitting and peeling nails. It is recommended to take such bath one or two times a week.

Ingredients:
- *1 part of ACV (for example 1 tsp.);*
- *1 part of warm vegetable oil (for example 1 tsp.).*

How to proceed:

- Thoroughly mix ACV and warm vegetable oil in equal proportions.

- Soak your nails in this bath for 10 minutes.

- Dry your nails well with a towel or paper napkin.

- Apply nourishing cream with gentle massaging moves.

BATH WITH ACV TO CURE SPLITTING AND PEELING NAILS

This baths helps to strengthen fragile nails and fights against splitting and peeling nails. It is recommended to take such bath one or two times a week. You can do it daily to achieve speedy results.

Ingredients:
- *2 tbsp. of ACV;*
- *100 grams of dried camomile flowers;*
- *2 cups of boiling water;*
- *1 tbsp. of sea salt.*

How to proceed:
- Take 100 grams of dried camomile flowers and place this into your teapot (you also can use a cafetiere or tea infuser).

- Pour 2 cups of boiling water into the pot and let it steep for 20-30 minutes.

- Strain the infusion into a suitable container.

- Add 2 tbsp. of ACV.

- Add 1 tbsp. of sea salt.

- Mix it all well.

- Soak your nails in this bath for about 10-15 minutes.

- Do not rinse.

- Dry with a towel or paper napkin.

- Apply your favourite nail/hand cream.

HAIR CARE RECIPES

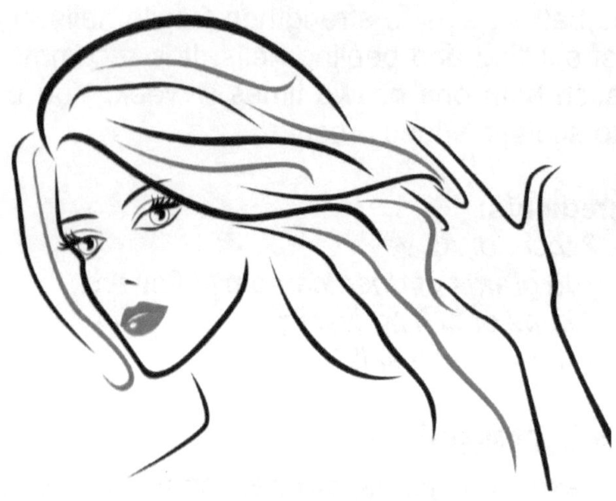

Natural apple cider vinegar helps to improve the condition of the hair and scalp by removing dandruff, eliminating itchiness to the scalp, normalizing oily scalps, making hair strong, soft, shiny and silky, and facilitating hair combing.

HAIR RINSING

Rinsing the hair with a solution of water and ACV very positively affects the condition of any hair type: hair is becoming shinier, silky, soft, strong, and easy to comb. Such rinsing can easily replace any hair conditioner. Do not worry that you hair will smell of ACV. Although it may be strong at the beginning, the ACV odor quickly disappears in the open air.

Ingredients:
- *3-4 tbsp. of ACV;*

o   *1 liter of water (it is better to use boiled water as it is softer).*

How to proceed:

- Dilute ACV in water.
- After washing rinse your hair with this solution.
- Do not wash off.
- Wring out the hair slightly and wrap with a towel.
- Air dry your hair at room temperature.

<u>Advices</u>:

- Do not use a hairdryer as it strongly dehydrates the hair.
- You can also add various herbal infusions to an ACV solution: chamomile will give your hair a golden tint, rosemary and nettle – maroon, and salvia (actively strengthens hair roots) – ashy.

RINSING FOR SOFT AND OBEDIENT HAIR

This rinsing helps your hair become softer and obedient. It is recommended to use this rinse one or two times per week.

Ingredients:
- *1 tbsp. of ACV;*
- *1 tsp. of fresh lemon juice;*
- *1 liter of warm water (it is better to use boiled water as it is softer).*

How to proceed:

- Dilute ACV and lemon juice in warm boiled water.

- Rinse your hair with this solution immediately after washing.

- Do not rinse off.

- Towel dry the hair at room temperature.

MASK TO IMPROVE HAIR CONDITION

This mask highly improves the hair condition. Your hair will become stronger, softer and gain a healthy beautiful shine. It is recommended to use this mask one or two times per week.

Ingredients:
- *2 tbsp. of ACV (for dry and normal hair) or 4 tbsp. of ACV (for oily hair);*
- *1 apple;*
- *1 egg yolk.*

How to proceed:
- Peel 1 apple, grate it or run it through a blender.
- Add 1 egg yolk and ACV.
- Mix it all together thoroughly.
- Apply the mixture to your clean wet hair.
- Wrap your head with polyethylene (plastic food wrap) and a towel.
- Wait for between 30 to 60 minutes.
- Wash the mask off with warm water.
- Air dry your hair at room temperature without using a hairdryer as this strongly dehydrates the hair, depriving it and your scalp of life-giving moisture.

RESTORING HAIR MASK

This restoring mask provides lots of benefits to the hair: they become healthier, stronger, shinier, and softer. It is recommended to use this mask one to two times per week.

Ingredients:
- *1 tsp. of ACV;*
- *1 tbsp. of honey;*
- *½ cup of water.*

How to proceed:

- Thoroughly mix all the ingredients together.

- Apply this mask to wet hair and scalp.

- Wrap your head with polyethylene (plastic food wrap) and a towel.

- Wait for about 1.5 hours.

- Wash the mask off with warm water.

- Air dry your hair at room temperature without using a hairdryer as this strongly dehydrates the hair, depriving it and your scalp of life-giving moisture.

ACV AGAINST DANDRUFF

<u>Recipe # 1:</u>

This procedure eliminates dandruff and also improves the blood circulation to the scalp, strengthens the hair roots, reduces hair loss, improves hair condition, makes it healthier and shinier and speeds up growth.

Ingredients:
- *Undiluted ACV (approx. 1 tbsp.).*

How to proceed:
- Rub undiluted, natural ACV into the hair roots for between 5 and 10 minutes before each hair washing.

<u>Recipe # 2:</u>

It is recommended to carry out this procedure one or two times per week. You will notice a positive effect even after two or three procedures.

Ingredients:
o   *Undiluted ACV (approx. 1 tbsp.).*

How to proceed:
- Slightly warm up undiluted natural ACV and apply it evenly to your scalp.

- Put on a shower cap and wrap your head with polyethylene (plastic food wrap) and then wrap your head with a terry towel.

- Wait for 1 hour.

- Wash your hair with your favorite shampoo.

- Rinse your hair with an ACV solution: 3-4 tbsp. of ACV + 1 liter of clean water at a comfortable temperature.

- Do not rinse your hair and do not use a hairdryer, let the hair air dry at room temperature.

<u>NOTES</u>:
- Prevent ACV from getting into your eyes. If this happens gently flush your eyes with clean cool water.
- You may feel a strong heat or even a slight burning in your scalp after applying ACV applying – this is a normal reaction, but if you experience an unpleasant feeling, rinse the ACV off with clean warm water and in the future always dilute it with water in a proportion optimal for you.

FOR DRY SCALP

If you have a very dry scalp which itches after each washing, try this recipe. This procedure decreases scalp itching, and long-term, regular use eliminates it at all. Repeat this procedure one or two times a week.

Ingredients:
- *3 tsp. of ACV;*
- *3 tbsp. of clean water.*

How to proceed:
- Mix ACV and water.
- Dip your comb or brush (It is better to use one with natural bristle) into an ACV solution and gently comb your hair until your scalp and hair become wet.
- Do not rinse.
- Do not wipe the hair and do not use a hairdryer – let your hair air dry at room temperature.

RECIPE TO PREVENT HAIR LOSS

If you carry out this procedure regularly, your hair will greatly benefit; the roots will become stronger as ACV actively improves blood circulation to the scalp; hair loss will be reduced and the hair itself will gain a healthier and beautiful appearance. It is recommended to repeat this procedure one or two times per week (better in the evening).

Ingredients:
- *1 part of ACV (for example 1 tsp.);*
- *1 part of clean water (for example 1 tsp.).*

How to proceed:

- Mix ACV and water in 1:1 proportion.

- Moisten your comb or brush (It is better to use one with natural bristle) with an ACV solution and massage your scalp for between 10 and 15 minutes.

- Do not rinse your hair. Don't worry that your hair will have smell of ACV as the odor quickly disappears in open air.

<u>NOTE</u>: If you have sensitive skin and feel a strong burning sensation during the procedure, add extra water in the solution: 1 part of ACV + 2 parts of water.

MASK FOR OILY HAIR

This effective apple mask helps to eliminate excessive greasiness to the hair, nourishes with useful vitamins and micronutrients and gives your hair an amazing shine and softness. It is recommended to use this mask once per week.

Ingredients:
- *1-2 tbsp. of ACV (depending on your hair length and your scalp sensitivity);*
- *apples (Depending on the length of your hair, use the following amount of medium sized apples. For short hair – two apples. For medium hair – four apples. For long hair – six apples);*
- *1 tbsp. of fresh lemon juice.*

How to proceed:
- Peel the apples, grate them or run them through a blender.
- Add ACV and fresh lemon juice and mix it all together thoroughly.
- Apply the mass evenly to all your hair and scalp.
- Wrap your hair with plastic wrap and a towel.
- Wait for 20-30 minutes.
- Wash off with warm water and your usual shampoo.

MASK FOR DRY HAIR

This mask has a powerful curative effect on the dry hair, improving its internal and external condition. It is recommended to use this mask one or two times per week.

Ingredients:
o   *1 tbsp. of ACV;*
o   *1 egg yolk;*
o   *1 tbsp. of castor oil.*

How to proceed:

- Thoroughly mix all the ingredients together.

- Rub this mask into the hair roots.

- Wrap your head with polyethylene (plastic food wrap) and a towel.

- Wait for one hour.

- Wash off with warm water and your usual shampoo.

MASK FOR BRITTLE HAIR

This mask actively strengthens the hair, making it less brittle, and gives your hair an amazing shine and softness. It is recommended to use this mask once per week.

Ingredients:
- *1 tbsp. of ACV;*
- *1 middle sized onion;*
- *1 garlic;*
- *1 tbsp. of kefir or Greek yogurt;*
- *1 tbsp. of honey.*

How to proceed:
- Grate one middle sized onion.
- Chop one garlic.
- Mix onion and garlic with kefir/Greek yogurt.
- Add honey and ACV and thoroughly mix all the ingredients together.
- Apply this mixture onto your hair and scalp.
- Wrap your head with polyethylene (plastic food wrap) and a towel.
- Wait for 1.5 to 2 hours.
- Wash the mask off with warm water and your usual shampoo.
- Rinse your hair with an ACV solution: 1 tbsp. of ACV + 1 liter of water at a comfortable temperature

NOTE: Do not worry that your hair will smell of onion or garlic as after you wash the mask off with a shampoo and rinse it with ACV solution, the smell will disappear.

MASK FOR HAIR GROWTH (FOR ANY HAIR TYPE)

This mask effectively stimulates hair growth making it stronger and healthier.

Ingredients:
- *1 tbsp. of ACV;*
- *1 tbsp. of castor or burdock oil;*
- *1 tbsp. of fresh lemon juice;*
- *1 egg yolk.*

NOTE: If you have long hair double the ingredients.

How to proceed:
- Mix all the ingredients thoroughly.
- Evenly apply on your wet clean hair and scalp.
- Wrap your head with polyethylene (plastic food wrap) and a towel.
- Wait for 30-60 minutes.
- Wash off with a suitable shampoo for your hair type.
- Rinse your hair and scalp with an ACV solution (3-4 tbsp. of ACV + 1 liter of water).
- Wring your hair slightly and then wrap it with a towel.
- Do not use a hairdryer. Let your hair air dry at room temperature.

REVITALISING SHAMPOO FOR ANY HAIR TYPE

This shampoo makes your hair strong, soft, and shiny.

Ingredients:
- *1 tbsp. of ACV;*
- *1 tbsp. of your favorite shampoo;*
- *1 tbsp. of castor or burdock oil;*
- *1 tbsp. of honey;*
- *1 egg yolk;*
- *2 tbsp. of water.*

NOTE: If you have long hair double the ingredients.

How to proceed:
- Mix all the ingredients thoroughly and froth it up.
- Evenly apply the mixture on your wet hair and scalp.
- Gently massage your scalp and hair for between 2 and 3 minutes.
- Wash it off thoroughly.
- Rinse your scalp and hair with water + ACV (3-4 tbsp. of ACV + 1 liter of water).
- Wrap your head in a towel.
- Do not use a hairdryer and let your hair air dry at room temperature.

SPRAY WITH ACV
FOR EASY TO BRUSH/COMB HAIR

Your hair will become more silky, shiny, soft to the touch, easy to comb, and obedient. You can use such spray daily.

Ingredients:
- *2 tbsp. of ACV;*
- *250 ml of clean water.*

How to proceed:
- Mix ACV and water.
- Pour this mixture into a suitable spray bottle.
- Shake well before use.
- Apply evenly on your hair.
- Let the hair dry at a room temperature.
- Comb or brush your hair as usual.

Warning: Do not brush or comb the wet hair, it damages them a lot, dry them first.

Advice: You can also add a couple of drops of your favourite essential oil to add a fragrance and boost the benefits of the spray. Lemon, citronella, bergamot, tea tree, mint, melissa, cedar, cypress, pine, and eucalyptus are great for oily hair. The dry hair love ylang-ylang, tangerine, orange, incense, lavender, patchouli, myrrh, and palmarosa. Camomile, sandalwood, aniba rosaeodora, vetiver, and geranium heal split ends and damaged hair. Rosemary, calamus, petitgrain, coriander, verbena, bai are good against hair loss.

ACV ORAL ADMINISTRATION TO BOOST YOUR ENERGY AND VITALITY AND IMPROVE THE CONDITION OF YOUR HAIR AND SKIN

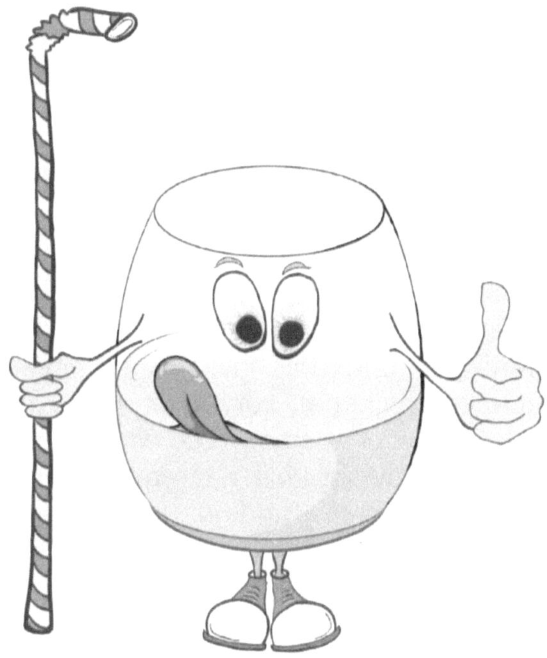

ACV oral intake is a powerful way to increase the vitality, strengthen the immunity, reduce sugar cravings and improve the condition of hair and skin. It also speeds up the metabolism helping to burn fat fast. ACV is often positioned as an effective means for weight loss, but be aware that if you have high levels of stomach acid, you should consult with a doctor before commencing an ACV oral intake.

It is possible to drink the diluted ACV one to three times a day. It should be taken for 30-40 minutes before a meal or at least an hour and a half after a meal.

Dilute two incomplete teaspoons of natural ACV into a glass (200-250 ml) of clean room temperature water, mix it well and drink slowly, taking small mouthfuls at a time. To improve the taste of the drink and to boost its healing effect, you can add one teaspoon of honey. However, it is not recommended to do this in the evening since the honey provides additional calories. It is better to use a drinking straw as this helps to protect your teeth enamel against ACV acids, or rinse your mouth thoroughly after drinking an ACV solution.

It is recommended to drink the diluted ACV for at least 30 minutes before a meal to allow the beverage to digest. It is also possible to drink it after a meal, but after an hour and a half to two hours to avoid ACV mixing with undigested food in your stomach (the rules of Hay Diet).

After starting to drink this invigorating beverage with natural apple cider vinegar, very soon you will notice an improvement in your body. You will become more vigorous, sugar cravings will decrease, and your hair and skin will gain a healthy and beautiful appearance.

CONCLUSION

In conclusion I would like to thank you once again for your interest in this book and for purchasing it.

In order to determine which recipes suit you best and effect your hair and skin in the most beneficial way, try one to two new recipes every week or two and watch your skin and hair condition. In this way after one to two months you will be able to choose an optimal collection of health and beauty recipes using ACV. I also recommend renewing this collection periodically (every 2-3 months) and trying other new recipes, since our organisms get used and adapt to the environment changes quite quickly. New recipes will stimulate the organism for regeneration and improvement in a new way.

Do not become a fanatical ACV user. Try to keep the recipes in proportion and follow the rule of a happy medium. Periodically take a one month break after long-term use of the ACV recipes – it will stimulate your organism to react to these recipes in a positive way.

From the bottom of my heart I wish you health, love, happiness and harmony with yourself and with the whole world!

www.ingramcontent.com/pod-product-compliance
Lightning Source LLC
Chambersburg PA
CBHW031419250726
48656CB00002B/745